WRINKLES, REWRITTEN

A SKIN-DEEP GUIDE TO AGING GRACEFULLY

Copyright © 2025

All rights are reserved, and no part of this publication may be reproduced, distributed, or transmitted in any manner, whether through photocopying, recording, or any other electronic or mechanical methods, without the explicit prior written permission of the publisher. This restriction applies to any form or means of reproduction or distribution.

Exceptions to this rule include brief quotations that may be incorporated into critical reviews, as well as certain other noncommercial uses that are allowed by copyright law. Any such usage must adhere to the specified conditions and permissions outlined by the copyright holder.

Book Design by HMDPublishing.com

DEDICATION

For every person who has ever looked in the mirror and questioned their beauty.

For every heart that has felt disheartened by the passage of time, or discouraged by the way age touches the skin and reshapes appearance.

May this book remind you that aging is a living story etched with wisdom, courage, and resilience.

May you find grace in each line, gratitude in each season, and joy in the reflection that has carried you through it all.

ACKNOWLEDGEMENTS

I am deeply grateful to everyone who made this book possible. To my family and friends who supported my passion for skincare education, thank you for your encouragement and patience.

To my parents, who have always been my biggest supporters in anything I pursue in life, I love you both so much and hope to make you proud.

To my fiancé, you have inspired me to take new paths, reach for the stars, and be the best version of me. Without you, I would never have pursued my dream to write. I love you so much.

To my clients, colleagues, and community, your stories and questions have inspired many of the ideas presented in these pages. And to every reader who opens this book: thank you for allowing me to be part of your journey toward embracing skin health.

Table of Contents

Chapter 1. Aging Beyond Skin: A Life's Reflection.................. 6

Chapter 2. The Science of Skin Over Time 16

Chapter 3. The Accelerators of Aging 24

Chapter 4. What We Can Do: The Inside Approach............... 34

Chapter 5. What We Can Do: The Outside Approach 44

Chapter 6. Myths, Fears, and False Promises........................... 54

Chapter 7. Aging is a Privilege 64

Chapter 8. The Grace of Growing into Yourself 70

Glossary of Key Terms..74

Also by Ashlyn Vaughn.. 80

Closing Note... 83

About the Author.. 84

CHAPTER 1

AGING BEYOND SKIN: A LIFE'S REFLECTION

When we think of aging, many of us instinctively picture mirrors. The fine lines that weren't there yesterday. The way our skin seems a little softer, less elastic, or marked with freckles from summers past. New marks, scars, and overall appearance. For some, these are small, quiet changes. For others, they trigger an alarm, as though an hourglass has suddenly appeared before us, its sand slipping away grain by grain.

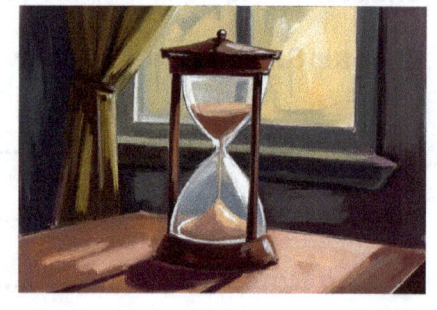

As a Skin Therapist, I have seen this from men and women time and time again. They often say skin aging came out of nowhere and they 'all of a sudden look twice their age'. Seeking the fountain of youth, these clients would request treatments and products to reverse the aging process.

Aging isn't only about what we see on the surface; it's the story of our entire lives written across our bodies. Each crease, freckle, and fold is an entry in the diary of living. We don't need to erase the writing, but we need to learn to read it in a different way.

Aging Through Time and Culture

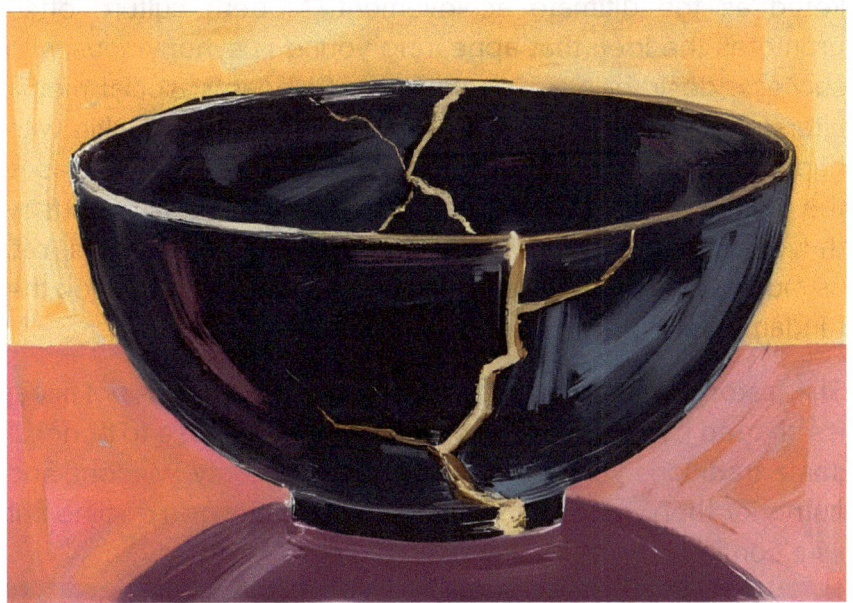

For centuries, various cultures have viewed aging with reverence rather than fear. In Japan, the practice of *wabi-sabi* honors the beauty of imperfection and impermanence. A cracked tea bowl, carefully repaired with golden lacquer, becomes more valuable due to its history. Wrinkles, too, can be seen as golden lines, proof of a life endured, cherished, and whole.

In many Indigenous traditions, elders are revered as living repositories of knowledge. Their weathered faces and hands are considered a map of wisdom, not flaws to be hidden. In parts of West Africa, gray hair has long been viewed as a mark of respect and authority. Ancient Chinese philosophy also placed value on aging, with Confucian teachings emphasizing filial piety and reverence for elders as a cornerstone of harmony. In India, the later stages of life are seen as a spiritual season—a time when detachment from material pursuits allows one to focus on wisdom, teaching, and inner peace. Even in ancient Rome, philosophers wrote of age as the season when perspective deepens and character shines most clearly.

Contrast this with much of today's world, where youth is marketed as the ultimate achievement. Modern culture often promotes the idea that appearing young is synonymous with success, desirability, and relevance. Billboards, social media filters, and glossy magazine covers equate smooth skin with happiness and vitality, creating a narrow standard that erases the dignity of aging. The multi-billion-dollar anti-aging industry thrives on that fear, offering quick fixes and miracle claims. Yet, as much as we try to resist it, no serum or surgery can undo the fundamental truth: time always moves forward.

Still, history reminds us that our perception of aging is not fixed; it's shaped by culture, values, and what we choose to honor. If some traditions view age as a symbol of beauty, wisdom, and authority, then we too can reimagine aging not as a decline but as a continuation of life's artistry.

> *"The key to both [wisdom and great tea] is proper aging"*
> *~ "Uncle Iroh" Avatar the Last Airbender*

Personal Mirror Moment

I remember the first time I leaned into the mirror and noticed faint lines on my forehead that didn't fade, even when my brows were at rest. For a moment, panic set in—*Oh no, here it begins.* I rubbed at my skin, hoping to smooth the lines away. But then I paused and thought of all the joy I've felt, the jokes I've told, the surprises that lifted my brows and etched these marks into place. That realization softened the moment: my skin wasn't betraying me, it was recording a life that had been lived fully.

Do I still catch myself checking the mirror, or trying to relax my brows so the lines don't deepen? Absolutely. Have I chosen to get a little Botox here and there? Yes. Did I need it? No. Do I regret it? Not at all. For me, caring for my skin is about support, not denial. I cleanse, I protect, I hydrate, but I've learned not to fight every sign of change. The truth is, there's no undoing the life experiences that shape us, and I wouldn't trade them for smoothness without story.

Skin as a Diary of Living

Your skin is more than a covering; it's a storyteller, carrying a living archive of your days. Every freckle and sunspot remembers summers of exploration, vacations by the sea, or afternoons spent tending a garden. Laugh lines are souvenirs of joy, evidence of countless smiles shared with friends, family, or even strangers who brightened a moment. 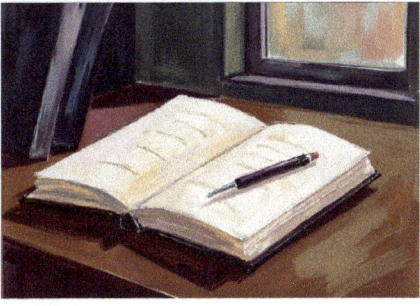 The small vertical creases above the lips may carry the memory of animated conversations, stolen kisses, or moments of fierce focus when life demanded your full attention. Even scars hold space as indelible chapters, testaments to challenges endured, lessons learned, and resilience proven.

Stretch marks whisper of growth. Bodies expanding to make room for new life, or shifting with the natural tides of change. Frown lines may reflect seasons of worry, yet they also reveal your capacity to care deeply, to carry the weight of responsibility, love, or loss. Together, these markings form a biography written not in ink, but in texture and tone.

Seen this way, aging skin is not a betrayal but a record, a living manuscript of resilience, vulnerability, and the privilege of time. It reflects the depth of your experiences and the grace of having lived long enough to accumulate such treasures. When we shift our gaze from criticism to curiosity, we begin to see our skin not as something to battle, but as a diary worth cherishing.

Try this: picture a person you love who is much older than you, perhaps a grandparent, mentor, or teacher. When you think of them, what stands out? Is it the depth of their crow's feet when they smile? The warmth of their weathered hands? Chances are, the things you love about them are inseparable from the very signs of age that we're taught to resist in ourselves.

The Emotional Weight of Appearance

Of course, this perspective isn't always easy to hold. We live in a world where every image is polished, edited, or filtered into an illusion of perfection. On social media, flawless skin is often presented as effortless and ageless, creating an unspoken pressure to measure ourselves against unrealistic standards. A scroll through these feeds can feel like falling behind in some invisible race, where the prize is eternal youth, and the cost is constant self-doubt.

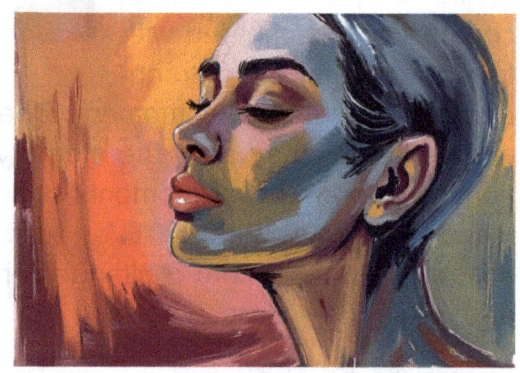

This pressure is heavy.
It can seep into the quietest parts of daily life: the pause before turning on a camera, the hesitation before stepping into good lighting, the sudden jolt when a candid photo reveals a side of ourselves we don't usually see. We're taught to chase after smoothness, symmetry, and sameness, as though the rich texture of individuality must be hidden away.

But no one gets through life untouched. If our skin never shifted, stretched, creased, or faded, it would mean we had not truly lived. That we had not laughed enough to carve joy into our cheeks, cried enough to soften the edges of our eyes, loved enough to wear tenderness into our expressions, or even stayed here long enough for time to leave its mark.

These changes don't make us less; they make us more. Each line, shadow, or shift is evidence of participation in the grand human story. They are proof of connection, of endurance, of the passage of seasons, and the persistence of spirit. Seen this way, our skin is a reminder that beauty is not about freezing time, but about embracing the life that time has given us.

Reframing Aging as Human, Not Cosmetic

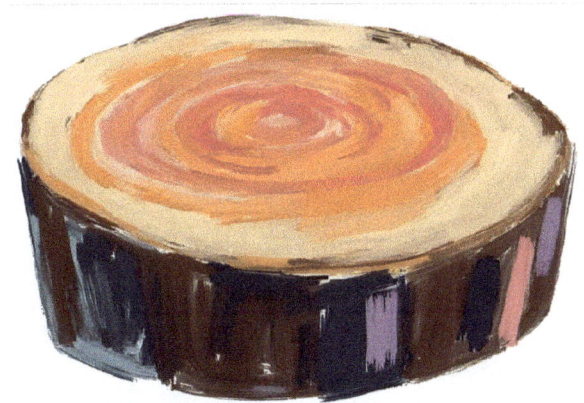

When we shift our lens, aging becomes less about what we lose and more about what we gain. Our skin, like the rings of a tree, grows and changes with each passing season. Each layer holds history, resilience, and transformation, reminding us that time leaves behind not emptiness but depth.

This book will not tell you how to stop aging, because that is neither possible nor the goal. Instead, it will help you understand how aging happens, what influences it, and how to care for your skin with knowledge, compassion, and confidence. It will offer tools to support your skin's health, while encouraging you to release the idea that every line or change is something to "fix."

Most of all, it will invite you to embrace the privilege of growing older, because not everyone gets the chance. To age is to continue the story. To age is to remain part of the world's unfolding. And to age with awareness is to claim beauty not as something slipping away, but as something evolving, chapter by chapter, with you.

Reflection Prompt

What's one wrinkle, freckle, or mark on your skin that reminds you of a happy or meaningful memory? Write it down here and celebrate the story behind it.

_____

_____

_____

_____

_____

_____

Timeline Activity

Draw a simple timeline of three milestones in your life, such as graduation, first job, becoming a parent, or any other defining moment. Beside each, jot down how your skin may have reflected that season.

Milestone 1: _____.

Skin reflection: _____.

Milestone 2: _____.

Skin reflection: _____.

Milestone 3: _____.

Skin reflection: _____.

Quiz

1. Your skin is compared to what in this chapter?
    a. A diary of living
    b. A battlefield
    c. A blank canvas
    d. A mask to hide behind

2. If your wrinkles could talk, what would they most likely say?
    a. "I'm proof you laughed, worried, and loved deeply."
    b. "You should've bought more serums!"
    c. "I'm here to ruin your selfies."
    d. "Nothing to see here."

3. Which culture celebrates imperfection and sees cracks as golden lines?
    a. Japan with the practice of *wabi-sabi*
    b. Ancient Egypt
    c. France during the Renaissance
    d. Modern Hollywood

4. When you think of someone older you love, what trait do you most admire?
    a. The depth of their smile lines
    b. Their wisdom and stories
    c. The comfort of their hands
    d. All of the above

5. What's the greatest gift of aging?
    a. Free birthday cake every year
    b. The privilege of continuing life's story
    c. Staying forever wrinkle-free
    d. Finally understanding how to fold fitted sheets

Answers:

1. ***a) A diary of living.*** Your skin isn't a battlefield. It's your biography. Every mark is a chapter.
2. ***a) "I'm proof you laughed, worried, and loved deeply."*** Wrinkles are storytellers, not enemies. Serums are nice, but stories are better.
3. ***a) Japan with the practice of wabi-sabi.*** Wabi-sabi reminds us that imperfection = beauty. A cracked tea bowl, a wrinkle, a scar are all golden lines of life.
4. ***d) All of the above.*** Chances are, what you love about them is inseparable from their age. Proof that aging adds, not subtracts.
5. ***b) The privilege of continuing life's story.*** Wrinkles may come with age, but so does perspective, love, and the chance to keep turning pages. (The cake is a bonus.)

CHAPTER 2

THE SCIENCE OF SKIN OVER TIME

Our skin may be the largest organ of the body, but it's also one of the most misunderstood. We notice when it changes—a new wrinkle here, a patch of dryness there—but most people don't realize what's happening beneath the surface. To understand aging, we need to understand the skin itself: how it is built, how it repairs, and how it transforms over the decades.

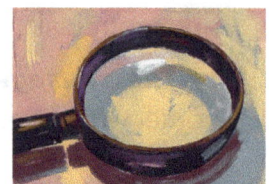

The Layers of Skin: More Than Meets the Eye

Skin is not just a surface; it's a living fabric, woven from layers that work in harmony. Each has a purpose, and together they protect, renew, and respond to the world around us.

The Epidermis: The Shield

This is the outermost layer, the surface we see when we look in the mirror. It's made of tightly packed skin cells, layered like protective tiles. Between these "tiles" are natural oils and lipids—the mortar—that seal in moisture and block harmful intruders. Every twenty-eight to forty days, the epidermis renews itself, shedding old cells and replacing them with new ones. As we age, this renewal process slows, which is why our skin may look dull or feel rougher over time.

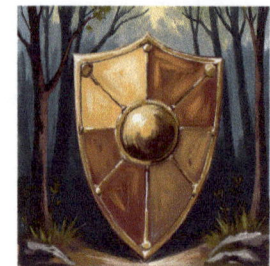

The Dermis: The Support
Beneath the surface lies the dermis, a framework filled with collagen (the protein that gives skin structure), elastin (which allows it to stretch and bounce back), and hyaluronic acid (which keeps it hydrated and plump). This is the layer that gives skin its strength and youthful resilience. Over time, collagen breaks down, elastin fibers weaken, and hyaluronic acid diminishes, leading to sagging and wrinkles.

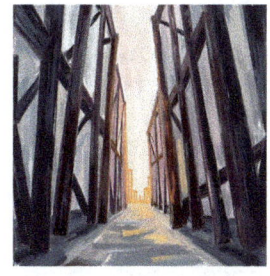

The Subcutaneous Layer: The Cushion
The deepest layer is composed mainly of fat and connective tissue. It acts like a soft foundation beneath the skin, providing contour and insulation. As we age, this layer thins, especially in the face, which is why the cheeks may appear less full and the skin can seem looser.

Together, these layers form a remarkable, breathing fabric that repairs itself, adapts to the environment, and quietly records the story of our years.

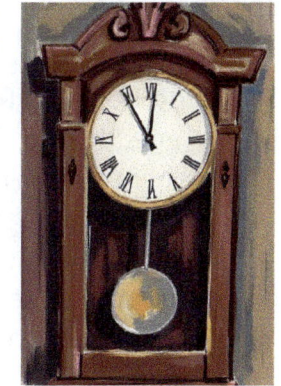

Intrinsic Aging: The Natural Clock

Certain aspects of skin aging are genetically determined. This is known as intrinsic aging—the natural, biological process that unfolds within us regardless of lifestyle choices. It's gradual, inevitable, and as natural as the heartbeat.

Slower Cell Turnover
In youth, skin cells renew quickly, rising from the lower epidermis to the surface in a smooth cycle of about twenty-eight

days. This rapid turnover keeps the skin luminous and resilient. With age, this cycle can extend to forty or even sixty days, allowing older cells to remain on the surface for longer periods. The result is skin that looks duller, feels rougher, and reflects light less evenly.

Collagen & Elastin Decline

Collagen—the protein scaffolding that gives skin its firmness—starts to decline as early as the mid-twenties, dropping about 1% per year. Elastin, which allows skin to stretch and spring back, also degrades. Imagine a mattress: when the springs weaken and aren't replaced, the surface loses its bounce. This is why fine lines deepen, cheeks lose fullness, and skin begins to sag.

Loss of Hyaluronic Acid

Another subtle change is the decline in hyaluronic acid, a naturally occurring sugar molecule present in the dermis. It acts like a sponge, holding up to 1,000 times its weight in water. With less of it, skin loses volume and hydration, contributing to dryness and a less "plump" appearance.

Hormonal Shifts

Hormones are key architects of skin health. Estrogen supports thickness and elasticity, progesterone regulates oil production, and testosterone influences collagen density. During menopause and andropause, the drop in these hormones accelerates visible changes: skin becomes thinner, drier, and more prone to wrinkles or sagging.

Reduced Repair & Regeneration

As we age, the skin's ability to repair itself slows. DNA repair enzymes work less efficiently, and antioxidant defenses weaken, so everyday stressors like UV rays or pollution leave a deeper impact. Cuts, blemishes, or sunburns take longer to heal. Over the decades, even small inefficiencies accumulate, manifesting as visible aging.

Intrinsic aging is universal. It's not a flaw or a failure, but rather a rhythm written into every cell, and it is proof that the body is following its natural design. While we cannot stop this process, understanding it allows us to care for the skin with more compassion, supporting its function rather than fighting its existence.

Extrinsic Aging: The Life We Live

While intrinsic aging is inevitable, extrinsic aging is influenced by our environment and lifestyle. These are the choices and exposures that can speed up or slow down visible changes. UV radiation, smoking, pollution, stress, poor diet, and lack of sleep all contribute to extrinsic aging. We'll dive into these factors in the next chapter, but for now, it's enough to know that extrinsic influences 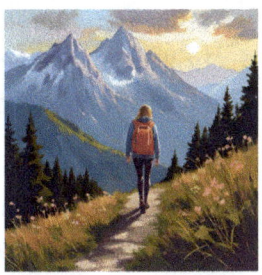 often account for up to 80% of visible skin changes.

This is why two people of the same age can look dramatically different. One person may have fine lines and sunspots, while another appears smoother and more evenly toned. Their genetics are the same age, but their environments and habits have left different marks.

The Decades of Skin

Skin doesn't change all at once; it evolves decade by decade. Understanding these shifts helps us both prepare and appreciate what's happening.

- **20s:** Collagen and elastin are plentiful, and cell turnover is fast. Most people enjoy naturally resilient skin, though early signs of sun exposure or lifestyle choices may begin to appear. Preventive care (especially sun protection) is key.

- **30s:** Fine lines may begin to form around the eyes and mouth. Collagen loss begins to show. Many notice uneven tone or texture. This is a decade when "prevention" begins to shift toward "maintenance."

- **40s:** Skin becomes noticeably thinner and drier. Expression lines settle into more permanent features. Hormonal changes may lead to acne flare-ups or changes in pigmentation.

- **50s:** Menopause and hormone decline accelerate skin changes. Skin loses its firmness, the cheeks may appear to hollow slightly, and sagging along the jawline often begins. Hydration and barrier support become critical.

- **60s and beyond:** Collagen and fat loss become more visible, and skin may bruise or tear more easily. Yet, there is also a softness and richness in texture that speaks to endurance. With consistent care, skin can still glow with vitality.

When Age Meets Practice

In my work as a skincare professional, I've learned that acknowledging the role age plays in skin health is essential when performing treatments or recommending products. For younger clients, oil glands are often more active, which can lead to congestion and breakouts if not appropriately balanced. For older clients, those same glands may slow down, leaving the skin drier and more fragile, and in need of nourishing oils and protective lipids.

This is just one example of how skin evolves. The key is to remember that skin doesn't stop working as we age; it simply changes tempo. Our job is not to fight against that rhythm, but to support it, adjusting our approach so the skin can keep moving in harmony with its natural beat.

Why Science Matters

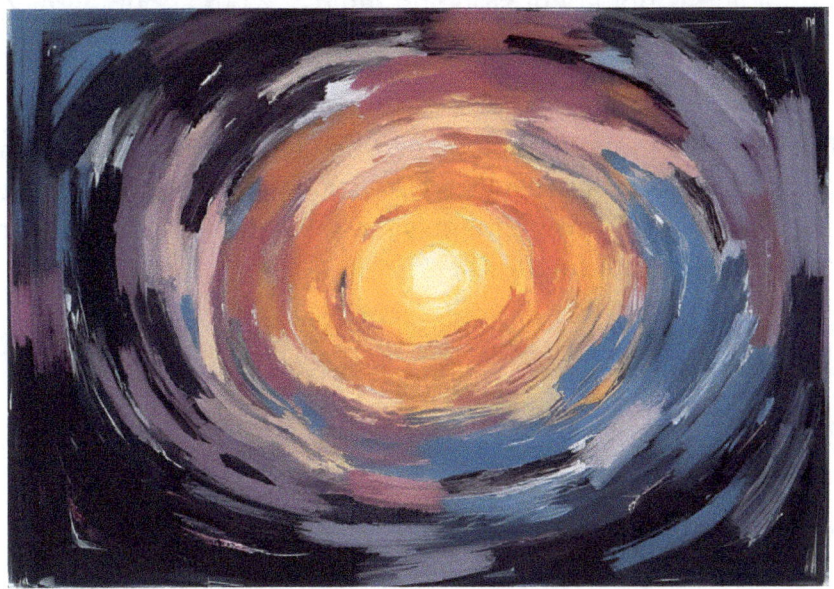

Understanding the biology of skin isn't just for dermatologists or estheticians. When you know *why* your skin changes, you can stop blaming yourself for looking older. Wrinkles aren't a punishment; they're the natural outcome of biology and life combined. Knowledge turns fear into acceptance, and acceptance is the foundation for graceful, empowered care.

Did You Know?

- Your skin accounts for about **16% of your body weight**.
- Blood vessels in the dermis stretch for **miles** in length.
- The skin renews itself about **1,000 times in a lifetime**. Though much slower as we age.

Bringing It Together

Skin is not static; it's dynamic, shifting, and alive. By understanding its layers, its natural rhythms, and its gradual changes, we can move into the next chapters with clarity. The journey of skin aging is not about *stopping the clock* but about learning how to work with time, protect what we can, and celebrate what we cannot change.

In the next chapter, we'll look at what accelerates aging—the choices and exposures that act like fast-forward buttons on the skin's timeline. Knowing them is the first step to making wiser decisions for your future self.

Quick Quiz

1. Skin cells renew every seven days.
   ❏ True   ❏ False

2. Collagen begins to decline in our 20s.
   ❏ True   ❏ False

3. Oil production increases as we age.
   ❏ True   ❏ False

Answers

1 = False

2 = True

3 = False

CHAPTER 3

THE ACCELERATORS OF AGING

Imagine two people, both fifty years old. One has smooth, resilient skin with only a few fine lines. The other has deeper wrinkles, uneven tone, and significant sagging. Their chronological age is the same, but their *skin age* tells a different story. Why is this?

The answer lies in the accelerators of aging. The choices, exposures, and environments act like pressing fast-forward on the skin's natural timeline. Unlike intrinsic aging, which is programmed into our DNA, these accelerators are primarily within our influence. Understanding them isn't about fear; it's about knowledge. When we understand what causes skin to age faster, we can adopt habits that help it age more gracefully.

Sunlight: Friend and Foe

We need the sun. It regulates our circadian rhythm, boosts our mood, and helps us produce vitamin D. Ultraviolet (UV) radiation is also the single biggest accelerator of skin aging, responsible for up to **80% of visible changes,** such as wrinkles, sagging, and dark spots.

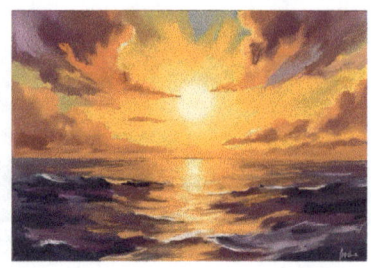

Here's what happens: UV rays penetrate the skin and trigger free radicals—unstable molecules that attack collagen and elastin fibers in the dermis. Over time, this weakens the skin's structure, like termites chewing through wood. UV exposure also stimulates excess melanin production, leading to pigmentation (those "sun spots" many of us notice in midlife).

Even short exposures accumulate. The fifteen minutes walking your dog, driving with your arm out the window, or skipping sunscreen on a cloudy day all add up. Dermatologists refer to this as photoaging, and it's the most preventable form of accelerated skin damage.

A Lobster on Easter Sunday

As an esthetician, I can tell you UV doesn't care if it's cloudy or cold. I learned this the hard way one Easter Sunday at a nearby lake. My family had rented a pair of jet skis for the afternoon. The weather was mild, with a light overcast, and the water was too chilly for swimming, so we brought no towels, no bathing suits, and most importantly, no sunscreen.

My sister and dad took one jet ski, while my mom and I climbed onto the other. It was my very first time on a jet ski, and it ended up being my last. A small hole in the machine allowed water to enter, and before long, we tipped over. Despite my years as a competitive swimmer, I panicked—near tears in a life vest—while my mom, who doesn't even swim, had to calm me down despite her own very real fear. (Mom, if you're reading this, thank you for your patience, and I'm sorry for the theatrics.)

We were stranded for nearly an hour before my dad was able to ferry us back to shore one at a time. By then, my mom and I were fried to a crisp, victims of one of the most memorable sunburns of my life. It wasn't even the worst burn I've ever had, but it was enough to turn me into a steamed lobster—all on a cloudy, breezy day when sunscreen never even crossed our minds.

That Easter etched the lesson into me forever: daytime SPF is non-negotiable, whether or not you can see the sunbeams.

Invisible Smog, Visible Impact

If UV light is a spotlight, pollution is the background haze that never quite goes away. Tiny particles from car exhaust, cigarette smoke, and industrial emissions are small enough to cling to the skin's surface, and some are so fine they can even penetrate deeper layers. Once there, they generate oxidative stress, releasing unstable molecules called free radicals. These free radicals chip away at healthy cells, weaken the skin's natural barrier, and trigger low-level inflammation that persists long after exposure.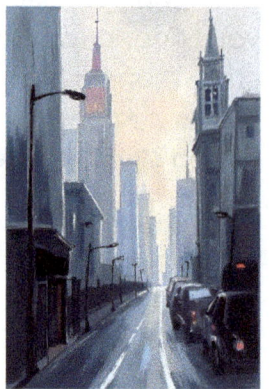

The skin does have its own defense system—antioxidants that neutralize these free radicals—but pollution steadily depletes them. Over time, this creates a cycle of vulnerability: the barrier becomes thinner, the skin grows more sensitive, and everyday exposures take a heavier toll.

Pollution doesn't just affect how skin feels; it accelerates the breakdown of collagen and elastin, the structural proteins that keep skin firm and elastic. It also disrupts the pigment-producing cells, leading to uneven tone and dark spots. This is why studies show that people living in urban or highly industrialized areas often experience more pronounced pigmentation and earlier visible signs of aging compared to those in rural regions.

Imagine your skin as a freshly painted wall. Each day, pollution acts like invisible smudges, scratches, and grit pressed against the surface. One mark may not be noticeable, but day after day, the wear accumulates, dulling the finish, weakening the structure, and leaving behind subtle but lasting changes.

The Daily Decisions Behind Aging

Some accelerators are less visible in the moment but carve deep marks over decades.

- **Smoking:** Nicotine restricts blood flow, starving the skin of oxygen and nutrients. Smokers often develop vertical lines around the mouth ("smoker's lines") and dull, sallow complexions.

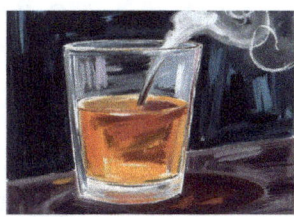

- **Alcohol:** Excess drinking dehydrates the skin, dilates blood vessels, and contributes to inflammation. Over time, this can lead to redness, puffiness, and broken capillaries.

- **Poor diet:** Diets high in sugar and processed foods contribute to glycation—a process where sugar molecules damage collagen, making skin stiffer and less elastic. Think of caramelized sugar hardening into brittle candy; that's glycation happening in slow motion under the skin.

- **Dehydration:** Without adequate water intake, the skin loses plumpness and becomes more prone to fine lines.

Stress and Sleep: The Silent Saboteurs

We often underestimate the extent to which stress is visible on our faces. Chronic stress keeps cortisol levels elevated, which breaks down collagen, slows healing, and increases oil production; a combination that can lead to fine lines, sensitivity, and breakouts. Stress also disrupts sleep, and without sleep, the skin loses one of its greatest tools of repair.

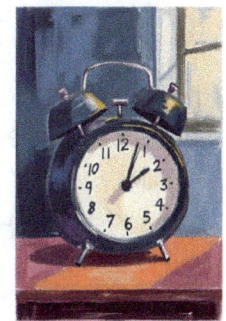

Nighttime is when the body shifts into "recovery mode." Growth hormone levels rise, supporting cell renewal and the repair of daily damage. Blood flow to the skin increases, delivering oxygen and nutrients that restore its glow. At the same time, the skin's barrier strengthens, preparing it to face the next day. When sleep is cut short, so is this entire cycle. The result can be seen almost immediately: dullness, puffiness, dehydration, and dark circles. Over the years, chronic sleep loss can lead to accelerated aging — from wrinkles to uneven tone.

Sleep and stress are deeply connected. When one is off balance, the other usually follows. Prioritizing both is not vanity, but biology: a way to protect collagen, preserve radiance, and give the skin the conditions it needs to do what it does best—repair, renew, and thrive.

The Weight of Exhaustion

I once worked with a client who confided, *"I feel like I've aged ten years in the past one."* She wasn't exaggerating. She was a nurse balancing long shifts, homeschooling her children, and volunteering with her church in the few hours left in her week. In hindsight, I don't know how she managed it all, but the constant stress showed on her skin, and more importantly, she *felt* it in every part of herself.

Her concern wasn't that her skincare routine had failed, but that her life had left her running on empty. The real accelerator wasn't a missing product; it was exhaustion. Together, we pared her routine down to the essentials so it felt doable, and we also shifted the focus of her professional treatments. Instead of just addressing surface concerns, we emphasized relaxation: dimmed lights, calming aromatherapy, gentle touch therapy, and soothing scalp massage. For her, those facials became a rare hour of stillness where her body and mind could rest.

Over time, that combination of simplicity and care made a visible difference. Her skin looked calmer, her eyes brighter, and she carried herself with a lightness that went beyond her reflection. It was a reminder that sometimes the most powerful skin treatment isn't about what we apply, but the space we create for the body to heal.

Inflammaging: Aging on Fire

A newer concept in dermatology and longevity science is inflammaging—the idea that low-level, chronic inflammation acts as a silent accelerator of aging throughout the body, including the skin. Unlike acute inflammation—the swelling, redness, and heat you see after a cut or sunburn, which signals the body's repair system is at work—inflammaging is different. It's a slow, smoldering process, often invisible on the surface, yet gradually breaking down the body's resilience from within.

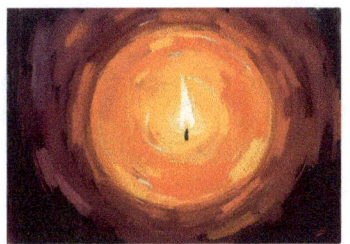

Many factors can fuel this type of chronic inflammation:

- **Lifestyle habits** such as high stress, poor sleep, and unbalanced diets.
- **Environmental exposures** like pollution, UV radiation, and toxins.
- **Underlying health conditions,** including metabolic or autoimmune issues.

Over time, this low-grade inflammation gradually erodes the very structures that keep the skin strong and supple. It accelerates the breakdown of collagen and elastin, slows wound healing, and increases skin sensitivity. Many visible signs of aging, such as thinning, sagging, dullness, or increased sensitivity, have roots in this subtle but persistent biological stress.

Inflammaging isn't just a skin concern; it's a whole-body phenomenon. The same inflammatory pathways linked to wrinkles and sagging skin are also associated with age-related conditions, including cardiovascular disease, diabetes, and neurodegeneration. In this way, the skin can serve as an outward indicator of deeper processes occurring within the body.

Taking Stock: Your Accelerators

Knowledge becomes power when we apply it. Reflect for a moment:

- Do you regularly wear SPF? Even on cloudy days or indoors near windows?

- Do you live in a city where pollution may be affecting your skin more than you realize?

- Do you smoke, drink, or rely heavily on processed foods?

- How many nights a week do you sleep fewer than seven hours?

- Do you notice stress showing up on your skin (breakouts, flare-ups, dullness)?

You don't need to eliminate every risk factor; no one can. But awareness gives you the freedom to choose where to focus. Often, small, consistent changes make the biggest difference in how skin ages.

> **Reflection Prompt**

Think of one accelerator that resonates most with your current lifestyle. Write it down, then jot one small, realistic change you could make this week to soften its impact. Perhaps it's adding SPF to your morning routine, opting for water instead of soda, or setting a bedtime reminder.

_____
_____
_____
_____
_____
_____

Empowered Decisions

Accelerators of aging don't exist to scare us; they exist to inform us. The good news? While we can't stop intrinsic aging, we can absolutely reduce the pace of extrinsic aging. Every mindful choice you make—a hat on a sunny day, a balanced meal, a full night's sleep—is a small gift to your future self.

In the next chapter, we'll explore exactly how to harness the *inside approach*: the foods, habits, and wellness practices that keep skin resilient from within. Aging gracefully doesn't start in a bottle; it begins with how we live.

Quiz

1. What do dermatologists call skin damage caused by years of UV exposure?
    a. Wrinkle-itis
    b. Sun-stamping
    c. Photoaging
    d. The lobster effect

2. 2. Which everyday habit can act like "caramelizing" your skin from the inside out?
    a. Eating too much sugar
    b. Drinking water
    c. Using sunscreen
    d. Smiling too much

3. Pollution affects skin by...
    a. Making it smell like exhaust
    b. Depleting antioxidants and causing oxidative stress
    c. Thickening the skin barrier to protect it
    d. Only dirtying the skin's surface (nothing more)

4. Stress and lack of sleep are called "silent saboteurs" because...
    a. hey secretly throw all-night parties without inviting you
    b. They quietly break down collagen and slow repair
    c. They only matter when you're young
    d. They don't affect skin at all

5. "Inflammaging" refers to...
    a. A skincare trend on social media
    b. Sudden breakouts after spicy food
    c. Chronic, low-level inflammation that accelerates aging
    d. The red glow after a workout

Answers:

1. **c) Photoaging.** Years of UV exposure = photoaging. The "lobster effect" (sunburn) is just the short-term drama!

2. **a) Eating too much sugar.** Sugar bonds to collagen in a process called glycation, like slow-motion candy-making in your skin.

3. **b) Depleting antioxidants and causing oxidative stress.** Pollution digs in your skin, stirs up free radicals, and messes with collagen and pigment.

4. **b) They quietly break down collagen and slow repair.** Stress and lack of sleep don't need to shout to leave a mark. They show up as dullness, dark circles, and lines.

5. **c) Chronic, low-level inflammation that accelerates aging.** "Inflammaging" = a slow fire inside the body. It's not a social media trend (yet), but it's definitely real biology.

CHAPTER 4

WHAT WE CAN DO: THE INSIDE APPROACH

We've seen how aging unfolds naturally and how certain factors can accelerate it. The empowering news is this: what you do from the inside out matters just as much—sometimes more—than what you put on your skin. Diet, movement, sleep, and emotional well-being all show up on your face in ways that topical treatments alone never can.

This doesn't mean striving for perfection. It means building a lifestyle that supports your skin the way good soil supports a garden. When the body is nourished, hydrated, rested, and cared for, the skin becomes a reflection of that inner vitality.

Nutrition: Feeding Your Skin from Within

Skin is not just a surface; it's a living, breathing organ that depends on the nutrients we provide it. Every bite of food contributes to the skin's ability to repair, renew, and defend itself. A balanced diet helps preserve collagen, calm inflammation, combat oxidative stress, and maintain a strong skin barrier that can withstand daily challenges.

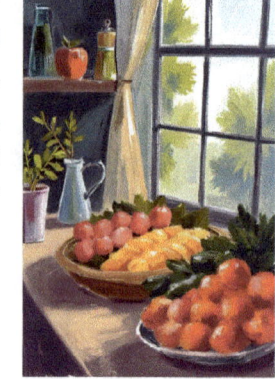

Antioxidants: Nature's Firefighters
Vitamins A, C, and E, along with

polyphenols found in colorful fruits, vegetables, and teas, act as the body's natural bodyguards. They neutralize free radicals before those unstable molecules can damage skin cells. Think of antioxidants as firefighters, constantly patrolling for sparks and putting out flames before they can spread. Diets rich in berries, leafy greens, citrus fruits, and green tea have been linked to brighter, more resilient complexions.

Healthy Fats: The Barrier Builders
Omega-3 fatty acids, found in salmon, walnuts, flax, and chia seeds, help maintain the skin's lipid barrier, which is the outermost shield that keeps moisture in and irritants out. Without enough healthy fats, the skin can become dry, rough, or more reactive. These fats also calm low-level inflammation, which supports a smoother, more even appearance over time.

Protein: The Building Blocks
Collagen, elastin, and keratin—the proteins that give skin structure, bounce, and strength—all depend on dietary protein. Eating a variety of high-quality sources, such as legumes, lean meats, tofu, eggs, and fish, provides the amino acids your body needs to rebuild and repair the skin continually. Without them, the skin heals more slowly and becomes more vulnerable to visible aging.

Hydrating Foods: Water + Minerals
While drinking water is essential, foods also play a vital role in hydration. Water-rich fruits and vegetables, such as cucumbers, melons, and leafy greens, deliver not only fluid but also essential electrolytes like magnesium and potassium, which help balance hydration at the cellular level. These foods help the skin maintain plumpness and softness from the inside out.

The Glycation Trap
On the flip side, diets high in refined sugar and processed foods accelerate **glycation**—a chemical process in which sugar molecules bind to collagen, making it brittle and less

elastic. Imagine caramelized sugar hardening into candy: the same stiffening effect occurs slowly under the skin, leading to wrinkles and a loss of suppleness. The good news is that small swaps matter. Choosing fruit over candy, or sparkling water over soda, can reduce this internal "stickiness" and protect your collagen for years to come.

Food doesn't just fuel the body; it sculpts the skin. Each meal is an opportunity to strengthen your skin's resilience, brighten its appearance, and support its natural defenses. What you put on your plate shows up in your reflection.

Exercise: Movement as Medicine

When your heart rate increases, blood flow improves, and with it, oxygen and nutrients reach the skin more efficiently. This is why people often describe having a healthy "glow" after a workout. That post-exercise flush isn't just a fleeting cosmetic perk; consistent movement supports long-term skin health by nurturing it from the inside out.

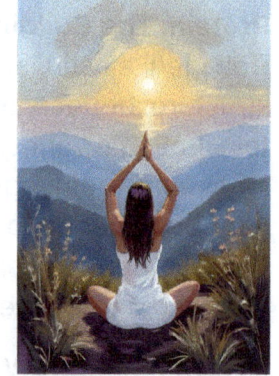

Improved Circulation
Exercise acts like a delivery service for the skin. With each heartbeat, fresh oxygen and nutrients reach the cells, while waste products are carried away more effectively. This renewed supply helps skin look brighter and function more efficiently.

Lymphatic Drainage
Beyond blood flow, gentle movement also encourages lymphatic drainage. The lymphatic system helps remove toxins and excess fluid from the body. Walking, stretching, or yoga acts like a natural pump, reducing puffiness and giving the skin a clearer, less congested appearance.

Collagen Support

Studies suggest that exercise reduces systemic inflammation, which accelerates collagen breakdown. By calming this "background fire" in the body, regular movement helps preserve collagen and elastin, the structural proteins that keep skin firm and resilient.

Hormonal Balance & Stress Relief

Physical activity also influences hormones in ways that benefit the skin. It lowers cortisol—the stress hormone linked to breakouts, sensitivity, and premature aging—while boosting endorphins, which support mood and overall well-being. When stress is lowered, the skin barrier can function more effectively.

Flexibility of Choice

Movement doesn't need to be extreme to make a difference. Walking, yoga, swimming, cycling, gardening, or even dancing in your living room all count. Gentle stretching alone increases circulation, keeps the body limber, and relieves tension, all of which are benefits that ripple outward into healthier, calmer-looking skin.

Exercise is more than a fitness goal; it's medicine for both body and complexion. Each time you move, you're not only strengthening muscles and heart health, but also giving your skin a natural, nourishing boost that no topical product can fully replicate.

Sleep: The Night Shift of Repair

We've all seen the evidence of too little sleep: dark circles, dullness, and skin that looks weary. But the truth runs deeper than a tired face. Sleep is not simply rest; it's when the body, and especially the skin, gets to work. At night, your

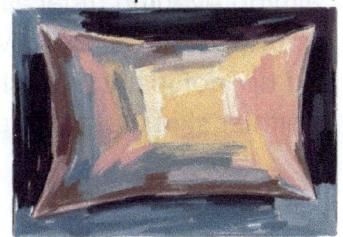

skin shifts into repair mode, tackling the day's damage and preparing for the next day.

Cellular Renewal
During deep sleep, growth hormone levels peak, stimulating tissue repair and the creation of new skin cells. This renewal process is what gives skin its vitality and helps fade the day's micro-damage from UV rays, pollution, and stress.

Barrier Strengthening
Overnight, the skin replenishes essential lipids—the natural oils that act as its protective shield. A well-rested barrier locks in moisture and keeps irritants out, making skin more resilient and less prone to dryness or sensitivity.

Inflammation Control
Sleep also helps regulate cortisol, the stress hormone known for breaking down collagen and thinning the skin over time. With adequate rest, cortisol levels stabilize, allowing the skin to maintain its firmness and elasticity.

The Cost of Sleep Debt
Chronic sleep deprivation accelerates visible aging in ways that skincare products alone cannot reverse. Collagen breaks down faster, wounds heal more slowly, and pigmentation or dullness persists for longer periods. Over time, the skin's ability to bounce back weakens, making the signs of fatigue look more permanent.

The Power of Consistency
Even small changes can create visible benefits. A consistent bedtime, reducing late-night screen exposure, or creating a calming evening ritual all help the body slip more easily into restorative sleep. Over weeks and months, these small habits add up, not just to a fresher face in the mirror, but to stronger, healthier skin that truly reflects rest.

No wonder the old saying calls it "beauty sleep." The phrase may sound quaint, but science confirms what tradition has long suggested: sleep is one of the most powerful, natural treatments for skin health we'll ever have.

Stress and Emotional Wellness

Stress isn't just a passing feeling; it's a cascade of chemical events that ripple through the entire body. When stress becomes chronic, cortisol—the body's primary stress hormone—remains elevated. Over time, this undermines skin health by increasing inflammation, weakening the barrier that keeps moisture in and irritants out, and accelerating the breakdown of collagen and elastin. What begins as tension in the mind eventually shows itself as sensitivity, dullness, or premature aging in the mirror.

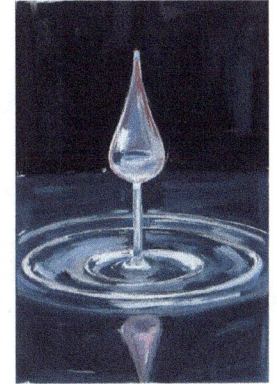

Emotional health, then, skin health. The two are inseparable. Just as the skin reflects the body's internal balance, it also echoes the state of our inner world. Prolonged worry, grief, or pressure can manifest as flare-ups of acne, eczema, or rosacea, while periods of calm and contentment often reveal themselves as radiance.

The encouraging part is that the same nervous system that reacts to stress also responds to intentional care. Mindfulness practices, such as meditation, journaling, or even taking a few slow, steady breaths, can help quiet cortisol and reset the body's stress response. These small acts don't have to be elaborate. Five minutes of stillness in the middle of a busy day can shift the body back toward balance.

Think of your skin as a mirror of your emotional state. A calm, cared-for mind radiates outward, softening expressions, easing reactivity, and giving the skin space to repair. When you nurture your inner world, your outer world often follows.

When Facials Weren't Enough

When I was in esthetics school, I imagined my skin would be the best it had ever looked. I was surrounded by products, learning professional techniques, and regularly practicing facials. If anything, I thought I'd graduate with the clearest, healthiest complexion of my life.

The reality was very different. I spent half the day in class and the other half working long shifts at a bakery. My "meals" were usually whatever was quick or free—endless cups of coffee, leftover pastries, and the occasional fast-food dinner scarfed down on the way home. Most nights, I managed only four or five hours of sleep before doing it all over again.

It didn't take long for the effects to show up on my face. Instead of glowing, my skin looked dull and uneven. Breakouts became a regular battle, and the dark circles under my eyes seemed permanent. It felt ironic. Here I was, surrounded by professional-grade products and treatments, yet my skin looked as close to the worst as it ever had.

Looking back, that season was my first real lesson in holistic skin care. Facials and serums can only go so far if the basics—sleep, nutrition, and stress management—are neglected. My complexion wasn't suffering from a lack of good products. It was suffering from exhaustion and imbalance. That experience shaped how I view skin health to this day: products are powerful tools, but they will never replace the foundation of taking care of the whole body.

> "Aging happy and well, instead of sad and sick, is at least under some personal control. We have considerable control over our weight, our exercise, our education, and our abuse of cigarettes and alcohol. With hard work and/or therapy, our

relationship with our spouses and our coping styles can be changed for the better. A successful old age may lie not so much in our stars and genes as in ourselves."
~George E. Vaillant

Lifestyle Swaps That Make a Difference

You don't need to overhaul your entire life to support your skin. Instead, focus on small, timeless habits that add up over the years:

- Drink a glass of water in the morning before coffee.
- Add one extra serving of colorful vegetables each day.
- Swap late-night scrolling for ten minutes of stretching or journaling.
- Step outside for natural light exposure in the morning to reset your circadian rhythm.
- Choose movement that you actually enjoy; consistency matters more than intensity.

Skin-Friendly Foods vs. Skin-Stressing Foods

Skin-Supporting Foods	Skin-Stressing Foods
Salmon, walnuts, chia seeds	Fried foods, trans fats
Leafy greens, citrus fruits, berries	Refined sugar, sweets
Green tea, herbal teas	Excess alcohol, energy drinks
Lean proteins, legumes	Highly processed meats
Cucumbers, watermelon, zucchini	Salty snacks that dehydrate

Reflection Prompt

Choose one inside-out practice to focus on this week. Maybe it's drinking more water, going to bed thirty minutes earlier, or adding a morning walk. Write down how you expect it might affect not only your skin, but also your overall mood and energy.

Beautiful Inside and Out

What you eat, how you move, rest, and manage stress all leave an imprint on your skin. These choices don't erase the passage of time, but they shape how gracefully it shows up. By nourishing your skin from within, you're not only protecting your appearance, you're supporting your entire body in aging with strength and resilience.

In the next chapter, we'll look outward to the rituals and treatments we apply directly to the skin. From daily cleansing and sunscreen to advanced professional care, you'll learn what truly makes a difference and how to avoid wasting time and money on empty promises.

Quiz

Match each accelerator to its effect on the skin.

A. Sunlight (UV radiation)
B. Pollution
C. Smoking
D. Alcohol
E. High Sugar Diet (Glycation)
F. Stress & Sleep Loss
G. Inflammaging

1. Restricts blood flow, causes dullness, and leads to vertical lines around the mouth.
2. Triggers free radicals that attack collagen/elastin, leading to wrinkles and sun spots.

3. Acts like caramelizing sugar under the skin, making collagen stiff and brittle.
4. Dehydrates the skin, dilates blood vessels, and contributes to puffiness and redness.
5. Tiny particles cause oxidative stress, weaken the barrier, and create uneven pigmentation.
6. Chronic imbalance raises cortisol, breaks down collagen, and disrupts skin repair.
7. Low-level, persistent inflammation that accelerates aging throughout the body and skin.

Answers:

1. **C. Smoking**. Nicotine narrows blood vessels, starving skin of oxygen and nutrients.
2. **A. Sunlight (UV radiation)**. The #1 cause of premature aging, aka, photoaging.
3. **E. High Sugar Diet (Glycation)**. Sugar bonds to collagen like sticky caramel, making it rigid.
4. **D. Alcohol**. Dries out skin and weakens capillaries over time.
5. **B. Pollution**. Creates oxidative stress, dullness, and dark spots.
6. **F. Stress & Sleep Loss**. Silent saboteurs that leave skin dull, puffy, and less able to repair.
7. **G. Inflammaging**. Chronic, "smoldering" inflammation that wears skin down over years.

CHAPTER 5

WHAT WE CAN DO: THE OUTSIDE APPROACH

So far, we've explored how the body and lifestyle shape the skin from within. Now, let's shift focus to the part most people think of first: what we apply on the outside.

The skincare industry offers an endless array of options for cleansers, creams, serums, and treatments. All promising youth in a bottle. It can feel overwhelming to sort facts from fads. The truth is, while not every product lives up to its claims, some approaches *do* have decades of science behind them. The key is learning what truly matters, so you can create a simple, timeless routine that works for you.

The Daily Essentials

Skincare doesn't need to be complicated. Three daily essentials are the backbone of every effective routine:

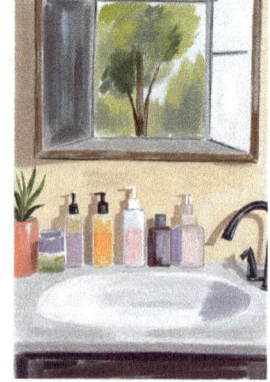

1. **Gentle Cleansing:** Removes dirt, oil, pollution, and makeup without stripping the skin barrier. Think of it as washing your favorite sweater: gentle enough not to ruin the fibers, but thorough enough to refresh.

2. **Moisturizing:** Replenishes water and lipids, helping the skin stay soft, flexible, and resilient. Moisturizers act like the sealant that keeps the "mortar" between skin cells strong.

3. **Sun Protection:** Sunscreen is the single most effective anti-aging tool available. Applied daily, it prevents photoaging (wrinkles, sagging, dark spots) more effectively than any treatment can reverse them.

These three steps—cleanse, moisturize, protect—remain relevant whether you're twenty or seventy. Anything else is optional support.

Ingredient Families That Stand the Test of Time

Instead of chasing the latest trend, focus on ingredients with proven longevity. Think of these categories as your "forever staples."

- **Retinoids (Vitamin A derivatives):** The gold standard for stimulating cell turnover and boosting collagen. They act like a personal trainer for your skin cells, encouraging them to renew efficiently.

- **Antioxidants:** Vitamin C, E, and other plant-based compounds help defend against free radical damage caused by the sun and pollution. Imagine them as tiny bodyguards patrolling your skin.

- **Peptides:** Short chains of amino acids that support collagen and elastin production. Think of them as construction workers, signaling your skin to build and repair.

- **Exfoliants:** Ingredients such as alpha-hydroxy acids (AHAs) or beta-hydroxy acids (BHAs) gently dissolve dead skin cells, restoring smoothness and radiance. Used correctly, they polish without sanding.

- **Barrier Protectors (Ceramides, Lipids, Hyaluronic Acid):** Reinforce the skin's natural wall against dehydration and irritation. These are the "mortar and glue" keeping bricks strong.

- You don't need every ingredient at once. Instead, think of your skin like a recipe: you can add or remove ingredients depending on your age, needs, and environment.

> *"Your skin is as unique as your fingerprints."*
> **~Jane Wurwand**

Professional Care: Beyond the Bathroom Shelf

For those who require additional support, professional treatments can deliver targeted results. They range from gentle and relaxing to advanced and corrective, with varying levels of strength, cost, and downtime. Each can play a role in a thoughtful "graceful aging" toolkit, but none are substitutes for daily care or overall wellness.

Facials

Professional facials are the foundation of skin maintenance. They go beyond what can be done at home, offering deep cleansing, exfoliation, hydration, and circulation support. Beyond the skin benefits, facials also provide a unique form of relaxation, lowering stress, calming the nervous system, and creating a space to simply *be cared for*.

Microneedling

This treatment uses tiny, controlled micro-injuries to stimulate the skin's natural healing response. In turn, collagen and elastin production are stimulated, resulting in a gradual improvement in firmness and texture. Think of it like aerating a lawn: by creating small channels, the skin is encouraged to regenerate with greater vitality.

Lasers
Laser therapies can target multiple concerns, from resurfacing rough texture to reducing sun damage, pigmentation, and fine lines. Some are gentle, requiring little downtime, while others are powerful enough to need days or weeks of recovery. All work by stimulating deeper repair processes and encouraging collagen renewal.

Chemical Peels
By applying controlled acids, chemical peels exfoliate the skin more intensively than at-home products. They can brighten dullness, smooth uneven texture, and refine tone, revealing fresher layers of skin beneath. The strength of a peel can be adjusted—from a light "lunchtime peel" to deeper treatments that require recovery.

Fibroblasting (Plasma Pen Therapy)

Fibroblasting is a non-surgical treatment that uses a plasma device to create controlled micro-injuries on the skin's surface. These pinpoint sparks stimulate fibroblast cells—the cells responsible for producing collagen and elastin. The result can include skin tightening, lifting, and improvement in fine lines and crepey texture, particularly in delicate areas such as the eyes or mouth. While results can be long-lasting, the treatment often requires downtime for healing, and it's not suitable for every skin type or tone.

Injectables (Fillers and Botox)
Injectables are among the most common professional options. Neurotoxins, such as Botox, temporarily soften expression lines by relaxing the underlying muscles, while fillers restore lost volume or enhance facial contours. This option may not be necessary for everyone, but for those who choose it, they can create subtle shifts that refresh without altering identity.

The key is to see professional treatments as support, not salvation. They can enhance, refresh, and complement your routine, but they cannot replace the fundamentals: consistent home care, sun protection, a balanced diet, adequate sleep, and effective stress management. Nor can they stop the natural rhythm of aging, and they shouldn't have to. Their actual value lies in helping skin function at its best and allowing you to feel more confident in your own reflection.

Everyday vs. Professional Care

Everyday Home Care	Professional Support
Gentle cleansing	Facials for upkeep
Daily moisturizer	Microneedling for collagen support
Broad-spectrum SPF	Lasers for pigmentation + resurfacing
Targeted serums (retinoid, antioxidant, peptide)	Chemical peels for texture + tone
Barrier care (ceramides, hyaluronic acid)	Injectables for temporary line/volume support

Separating Needs from Noise

Skincare shelves are overflowing with a multitude of choices: serums, masks, oils, mists, and various gadgets. Promises of "miracle" results fill labels, ads, and social media posts, each one suggesting you need just one more product to get it right, finally. Many of these items can be enjoyable additions, but they are not essential for healthy skin. To avoid overwhelm, pause and ask yourself: *Is this supporting my skin health goals, or is it just adding clutter?*

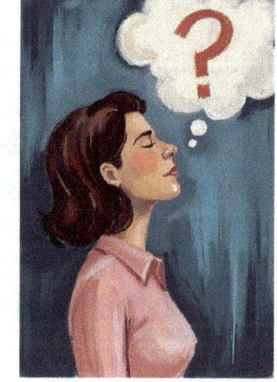

The truth is, your skin doesn't need twelve steps. What it needs is consistency. A handful of well-chosen, high-quality products—cleanser, moisturizer, and sunscreen as a foundation—will do more for your skin in the long run than a complicated routine that feels like a chore and gets abandoned after a month.

Complicated routines aren't just unnecessary; they can sometimes do more harm than good. Over-exfoliating, layering incompatible actives, or switching products too quickly can leave the skin confused, irritated, and less resilient. By focusing on *needs, not noise*, you protect your skin's natural rhythm instead of overwhelming it.

A skincare routine should feel like self-care, not homework. If a product brings you joy, adds a sensory ritual, or helps you feel grounded, it may be worth keeping, but only if it fits into a routine you can sustain. Ultimately, consistency, simplicity, and support will consistently outperform excess.

Building a Routine That Lasts

Aging gracefully isn't about chasing perfection; it's about creating rituals that feel doable, supportive, and even enjoyable. The best skincare routine is the one you can maintain, not just for a week, but for years to come.

A lasting routine is not built on pressure or guilt, but on rhythm. It should fit into your life as naturally as brushing your teeth or making your morning coffee. Some days may be more elaborate, with a mask or serum added for extra attention, while other days may be simple, just focusing on the basics. What matters is the steady beat of consistency, not perfection.

Skincare is also a conversation with your future self. Each time you protect your skin today, you are writing a thank-you note to the person you'll be in ten years. Those thank-you notes don't have to be long or complicated. They just have to be written, day after day, in the language of care.

Then skincare becomes less about resisting the signs of age and more about nurturing longevity. A self-care routine that lasts is about the relationship you build with yourself in the mirror: steady, kind, and enduring.

Finding Balance in the Sun

Some of the greatest changes I've seen in clients don't come from dramatic treatments; they come from small, sustainable shifts in their daily routines.

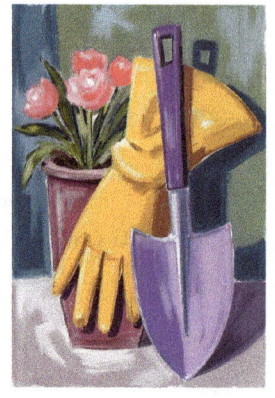

One client had been a faithful advocate for facials for years. She loved the way they made her skin look and feel, and she often left my treatment room glowing. But over time, she became frustrated. The results seemed to fade more quickly, fine lines deepened, and dark spots kept returning. She told me, almost in defeat, "I feel like I'm doing everything right, but my skin is still slipping backward."

Rather than pushing harder with more treatments, we stepped back to look at her everyday habits. That's when the real culprit became clear. She adored gardening; it was her joy, her therapy, her favorite way to spend hours outdoors. She often wore a wide-brimmed hat, but she couldn't stand the feel of sunscreen on her face. "It makes me sweat more, and it just feels heavy," she would say.

Together, we explored options. Limiting her gardening time wasn't realistic; it was something she loved too much to give up. Instead, we tried different formulas of sunscreen, focusing on lighter, more breathable textures. I also encouraged her to take small breaks in the shade when possible. After sampling a few products, she finally found one that felt comfortable enough to use daily.

The shift was subtle but powerful. She didn't have to give up her passion for gardening, and at the same time, her skin began to improve. Her results from facials started lasting longer, her dark spots began to fade, and she felt more in control of her skin health. What changed wasn't just her product, but her perspective: protecting her skin became something that fit into her life, rather than something that took away from it.

Reflection Prompt

Look at your current routine. Which steps feel essential, and which feel overwhelming? Write down one adjustment. Either add a key step (like SPF) or simplify by letting go of a product that doesn't serve you.

_____
_____
_____
_____
_____
_____
_____

A Partnership of Care

Skincare is not magic, but it's meaningful. The outside approach, when rooted in science and simplicity, works hand in hand with the inside approach to protect, strengthen, and celebrate your skin. Together, they form a partnership:

your habits on the inside fuel resilience, while your rituals on the outside provide defense and support.

In the next chapter, we'll shift gears to confront some of the biggest myths and fears about aging as well as explore how to spot false promises before they waste your time, money, and confidence.

Quiz

1. What are the three daily skincare essentials that matter at any age?
    a. Cleanser, moisturizer, sunscreen
    b. Toner, serum, face mist
    c. Clay mask, jade roller, sheet mask
    d. Eye cream, lip balm, overnight mask

2. Retinoids are often called the "gold standard" because they...
    a. a) Make your skin shimmer like gold
    b. b) Encourage cell turnover and boost collagen
    c. c) Hydrate the skin instantly
    d. d) Work best only in facials, not at home

3. Which ingredient family acts like "construction workers" signaling the skin to build and repair?
    a. Antioxidants
    b. Peptides
    c. Exfoliants
    d. Barrier protectors

4. Professional treatments can support skin health but which statement is true?
    a. They replace the need for daily SPF
    b. They can enhance results but don't stop natural aging

c. The stronger the treatment, the longer-lasting the results
   d. They're only for people over 50

5. What's the real secret to a routine that lasts?
   a. Buying every trending product you see on social media
   b. A 12-step ritual packed with actives
   c. Consistency and simplicity you can stick with long-term
   d. Never using the same product twice

Answers:

1. *a) Cleanser, moisturizer, sunscreen.* These are the timeless backbone of skincare. Everything else is optional support, not essential.
2. *b) Encourage cell turnover and boost collagen.* Retinoids train skin cells to renew efficiently. No glitter required.
3. *b) Peptides.* Like construction workers, they signal the skin to rebuild collagen and elastin.
4. *b) They can enhance results but don't stop natural aging.* Facials, lasers, injectables — they support you, but can't replace daily care or the passage of time.
5. *c) Consistency and simplicity you can stick with long-term.* Skincare works best when it feels like brushing your teeth, doable every day, not overwhelming.

CHAPTER 6

MYTHS, FEARS, AND FALSE PROMISES

The skincare world is full of hope and hype. Every year, new products, devices, and treatments are advertised as breakthroughs, each promising smoother, firmer, and younger-looking skin. Some of these have real science behind them. Many do not.

In this chapter, we'll strip away the confusion by looking at the biggest myths and false promises surrounding skin aging. The goal is not to shame anyone who has tried them—after all, curiosity is a natural human trait. The goal is to help you distinguish between what works and what wastes time, money, and peace of mind.

The Myth of "Anti-Aging"

"I am appalled that the term we use to talk about aging is 'anti.' Aging is as natural as a baby's softness and scent. Aging is human evolution in its pure form."
~Jamie Lee Curtis

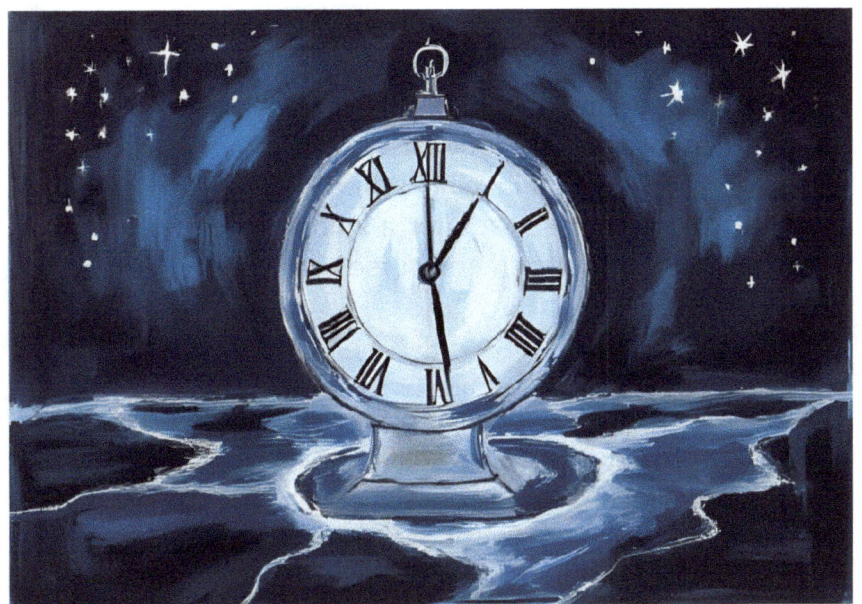

The very phrase *"anti-aging"* is misleading. Aging is not an illness to cure or an enemy to defeat; it's a natural, universal process that begins the moment we are born. Yet, for decades, the beauty industry has framed aging as something shameful to be resisted at all costs. The words themselves carry weight: "anti" implies that to grow older is a failure, and that youth is the only state worth striving for.

This language shapes our self-perception. It feeds fear, reinforces stigma, and makes people doubt their worth as soon as fine lines appear. The result is an endless cycle of chasing products that promise the impossible: to "reverse," "erase," or "stop" time. But nothing—no serum, procedure, or miracle ingredient—can halt the biological clock.

This doesn't mean we should neglect our skin or abandon self-care. It means we should approach products and treatments with honesty and clarity. Skincare can absolutely make a difference: it can slow the visible effects of aging, keep the skin comfortable and resilient, and help us feel more confident in our appearance. But its role is supportive, not oppositional.

Instead of "anti-aging," a better frame is graceful aging—caring for the skin as it changes, protecting it from unnecessary harm, and celebrating the marks of a life well-lived. The goal is not to erase the passage of years, but to move through them with health and comfort in mind. When we release the myth of "anti-aging," we make space for a kinder, more realistic relationship with both our skin and ourselves.

False Promises on the Shelf

The skincare industry is full of bold claims, shiny packaging, and buzzwords designed to spark hope and open wallets. Some promises recur repeatedly, creating cycles of excitement and disappointment. Let's look closer at a few of the most common myths.

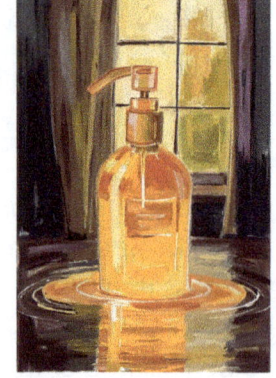

"Collagen Creams Replace Lost Collagen."
Collagen is one of the most important proteins in our skin, but it's also a very large molecule. Applied topically, it cannot penetrate the skin barrier to rebuild the collagen network beneath the surface. Creams labeled with collagen may still be useful, as they can hydrate, soften, and temporarily plump the skin's appearance. They don't actually *replace* what time has taken away. If the goal is to stimulate collagen production, ingredients like retinoids, peptides, and vitamin C—which can signal the skin to produce more of its own collagen—are far more effective.

"This Product Will Erase Wrinkles Overnight."
No topical product can permanently erase wrinkles overnight. What "miracle" creams often do is hydrate the skin, making fine lines appear softer until the moisture is absorbed. Some may include ingredients like silicones that create a smoother surface temporarily. These effects can be satisfying in the

short term, but they are not a true reversal. Lasting improvement comes from consistent daily care, patience, and, when desired, professional treatments that work more deeply in the skin.

"Natural Means Better."
"Natural" is a powerful marketing word, but it doesn't automatically mean safer or more effective. Poison ivy is natural. So is mercury. Meanwhile, many lab-created ingredients are both safe and highly effective, having gone through years of research and stability testing. Synthetic peptides, stabilized vitamin C, and hyaluronic acid are lab-born ingredients that benefit skin in ways many "all-natural" products cannot. What matters is evidence and formulation, not whether the source is from a plant or a lab.

"More Steps = Better Results."
The rise of multi-step routines has led some people to believe that more products equal more benefits. But layering too many formulas can backfire. It can increase the risk of irritation, barrier disruption, or even render active ingredients ineffective when they conflict. A simple, consistent routine of a few well-chosen products will consistently outperform a cluttered lineup abandoned after a month. Skincare is not about how many bottles sit on your counter; it's about how well you care for your skin day after day.

False promises thrive because they tap into a very human hope: the desire for quick fixes. But real skin health is built on honesty, science, and steady habits. Understanding what products *can* and *cannot* do enables you to make informed choices that save time, money, and frustration, while providing your skin with the care it truly needs.

The Influence of Fear

Much of the skincare industry thrives on fear. Fear of wrinkles, sagging, or being "left behind." Fear sells because it feeds on insecurity. Entire product lines are built on the suggestion that youth is slipping away, and that only a particular cream, serum, or device can rescue it.

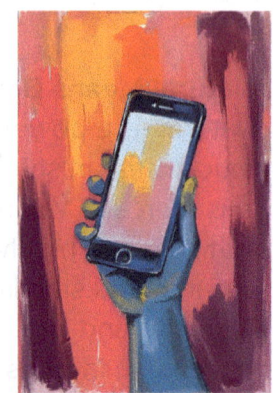

Social media magnifies this pressure. Filters smooth every line, retouching erases pores, and carefully staged lighting makes flawless skin seem effortless and real. The constant stream of "perfect" faces creates an impossible standard. It tells us that natural skin—with texture, pores, and changes over time—is a problem to fix. Before long, we start noticing "flaws" we had never worried about, simply because someone told us they were flaws.

But fear is not a sustainable motivator. Skincare driven by fear often leads to overwhelm: cabinets filled with unused products, routines abandoned in frustration, and a cycle of disappointment when "miracle" results don't appear. Worse, it can chip away at self-worth, making every new line or freckle feel like evidence of failure.

Skincare rooted in self-care feels different. It's not about punishment or erasing signs of age; it's about support, nourishment, and respect for the skin you live in. When the goal shifts from fixing to caring, the process becomes lighter and more empowering. Each step becomes less about battling the mirror and more about honoring yourself in the moment.

Ultimately, fear tells us we're not enough. Self-care reminds us we always were.

The Role of Trends and Fads

Every few years, a new "miracle" ingredient or device sweeps through the skincare world, promising dramatic transformations. One moment it's snail mucin, the next it's gold flakes in sheet masks, or at-home gadgets marketed as delivering "facelift-like" results. Social media accelerates these cycles, turning niche ideas into viral sensations almost overnight. Before long, products sell out, hashtags trend, and everyone feels the pressure to try the latest craze or risk being "left behind."

The truth is, most of these trends are fleeting. Some offer mild benefits. Snail mucin can be hydrating, and certain devices may give a temporary tightening effect. Yet, they rarely live up to the sweeping promises printed on their packaging. By the time the next big thing arrives, last year's "must-have" has often been forgotten at the back of a bathroom cabinet.

What remains consistent over decades is far less glamorous, but infinitely more powerful: daily sunscreen, a balanced diet, steady hydration, restorative sleep, and proven ingredients like retinoids, vitamin C, peptides, and niacinamide. These fundamentals may not be flashy, but they work.

This doesn't mean you can't enjoy trends. Skincare can be fun, sensory, and even playful. A trendy mask may feel luxurious, or a new serum may add excitement to your routine. But it helps to view trends as extras, not essentials—like accessories that complement an outfit, but don't replace the core wardrobe. When the basics are strong, you can experiment without getting lost in the noise.

The Cost of Chasing Eternal Youth

The pursuit of eternal youth often comes at a steep price and not just in dollars. Yes, skincare and cosmetic procedures can drain bank accounts, especially when every new launch is marketed as a "must-have" or every treatment is sold as the missing key. The heavier toll is often emotional.

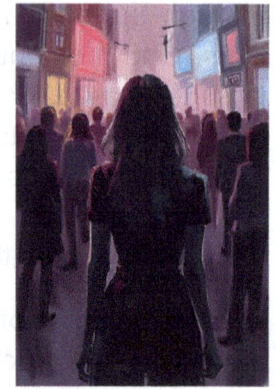

There is the disappointment of "miracle" creams that don't deliver, leaving yet another half-used jar on the shelf. There is the stress of scrolling through retouched images and feeling like you're always behind. There is the guilt of skipping steps in a ten-product routine or deciding not to splurge on the latest treatment. Slowly, these feelings chip away at self-worth, turning skincare from an act of care into a cycle of anxiety.

The deeper problem is that the chase has no finish line. Youth, by its very nature, cannot be preserved forever. So every attempt to freeze it sets up an impossible expectation. No matter how many products you buy or how many treatments you try, time will continue to move forward. When skincare becomes a race against the inevitable, the result is exhaustion, frustration, and disconnection from what skincare should be: support, not struggle.

The truth is, you don't need to buy every launch or follow every trend to age beautifully. What you need is a routine that feels sustainable, products that serve your skin instead of your fears, and the perspective to see beauty not as something slipping away but as something evolving. Peace of mind is, in itself, a form of beauty, one that no cream can sell you, but one you can cultivate when you step off the treadmill of chasing eternal youth.

Truth or Hype? A Quick Quiz

1. Collagen creams rebuild your skin's collagen.
2. Sunscreen is one of the most powerful anti-aging products.
3. More expensive always means more effective.
4. Stress can accelerate visible skin aging.
5. Natural products are always safer than synthetic ones.

Answers:

1. ✗ Hype. Collagen is a large protein, far too big to be absorbed through the skin. While creams may contain collagen or collagen-boosting ingredients, they don't rebuild your collagen directly. What they can do is hydrate, support your skin barrier, and sometimes stimulate your own collagen production if they contain proven actives like retinoids and peptides. But no cream can 'add' collagen back into your skin.

2. ☑ Truth. Nothing protects your skin from premature aging more effectively than sunscreen. UV rays break down collagen, create fine lines, dark spots, and uneven tone over time. Sunscreen is the most effective topical product to minimize UV damage.

3. ✗ Hype. A high price tag doesn't guarantee high performance. Many drugstore products use the same clinically backed ingredients as luxury brands. What matters most is the formula, not the label. A $20 retinol that's well-made can outperform a $200 cream without proven actives. Don't let marketing convince you that more dollars = more results.

4. ☑ Truth. Chronic stress raises cortisol. A hormone that breaks down collagen and elastin. Over time, this speeds up the formation of texture, dullness, and even breakouts.

Stress also disrupts sleep and self-care routines which are both essential for healthy skin. Managing stress with movement, mindfulness, or even good laugh can improve your skin.

5. ✘ Hype. "Natural" doesn't always mean "better" or "gentle." Poison Ivy is natural, but you wouldn't rub it on your face. On the flip side, many lab-made (synthetic) ingredients are safe, stable, and well-researched. As far as efficacy goes, the key is how an ingredients works with your skin, not where it came from. Safety depends on testing, concentration, and formulation.

Shifting From Fear to Facts

It's easy to feel discouraged when you realize just how much misinformation surrounds skincare and the aging process. From viral social media hacks to products marketed with exaggerated promises, the noise can feel overwhelming. However, knowledge is powerful and liberating. When you understand what's real, you can step out of the cycle of fear and confusion. You can stop wasting energy (and money) on gimmicks that prey on insecurity, and instead invest your time, effort, and resources into practices that truly support your skin.

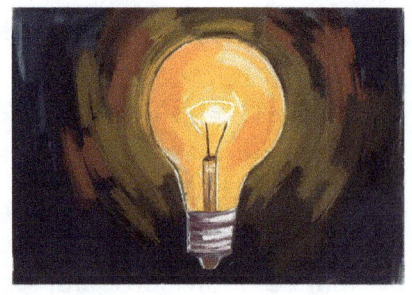

The real secret to aging well isn't hidden in a fancy jar; it's found in daily habits, science-backed ingredients, and the confidence that comes from embracing your journey.

Reflection Prompt

Think back to a product or trend you once tried that didn't live up to its promises. How did it make you feel? Now, imagine approaching skincare from a place of curiosity and care, rather than urgency or fear. How would that shift your choices?

_____
_____
_____
_____
_____
_____
_____

Heart Instead of Hype

Myths, fears, and false promises will always exist, but they don't have to guide your choices. When you replace hype with knowledge, skincare becomes simpler, calmer, and more rewarding.

In the next chapter, we'll explore the heart of this book: why aging itself is not a curse, but a privilege. We'll explore how each line, freckle, and change is a testament to a life lived and why the most powerful beauty secret is acceptance.

CHAPTER 7

AGING IS A PRIVILEGE

At some point in our lives, each of us has probably looked in the mirror and wished we could turn back time. The crease between our brows, the deepening crow's feet, the sag along the jawline. They can feel like reminders of something slipping away.

Here's the truth that we often forget: every line, every change, every shift in our skin is proof that we've made it this far. Aging is not a curse. It's a privilege denied to many.

The Gift of Longevity

When you view wrinkles solely as flaws, you miss what they truly signify. Laugh lines mean you've laughed. Freckles and sunspots mean you've spent days in the light. A silver strand of hair or softer jawline means you've carried decades of memories, love, challenges, and growth.

Consider those who never had the chance to grow older. Every year we live is a gift, and every mark of time is evidence that we are still here, still becoming.

Wrinkles as Storylines

Think of wrinkles not as cracks, but as storylines. The crow's feet that frame your eyes? Proof that you've smiled, squinted in the sun, maybe cried deeply when life demanded it. The folds that shape around the mouth? A record of countless conversations, kisses, and bursts of laughter. Even the loosening of skin around the neck and jaw shows the simple truth: you have lived, you have grown, you have endured.

In this way, skin becomes less about beauty standards and more about biography.

> *"Wrinkles should merely indicate where smiles have been."*
> **~Mark Twain**

Redefining Beauty

In cultures where elders are honored, beauty isn't seen in smoothness but in presence. The warmth of someone's smile, the sparkle in their eyes, the way their face softens with kindness. These qualities transcend time.

We're conditioned to fear aging because industries profit when we feel inadequate. But beauty is not erased with age; it's redefined. It shifts from being about symmetry and perfection to being about authenticity and spirit. True beauty is not the absence of wrinkles but the presence of life.

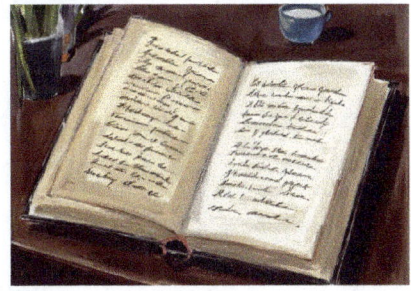

Reclaiming the Narrative

Aging gracefully doesn't mean neglecting yourself. It means shifting your narrative from fear to respect. You can still nourish your body, care for your skin, and enjoy the rituals of self-care, not because you're trying to erase time, but because you're honoring yourself through every season of life.

This shift changes everything. Skincare becomes an act of kindness rather than combat. Healthy habits become ways to enjoy life, not escape it. You stop chasing an impossible ideal and begin embracing the reality of who you are, right here, right now.

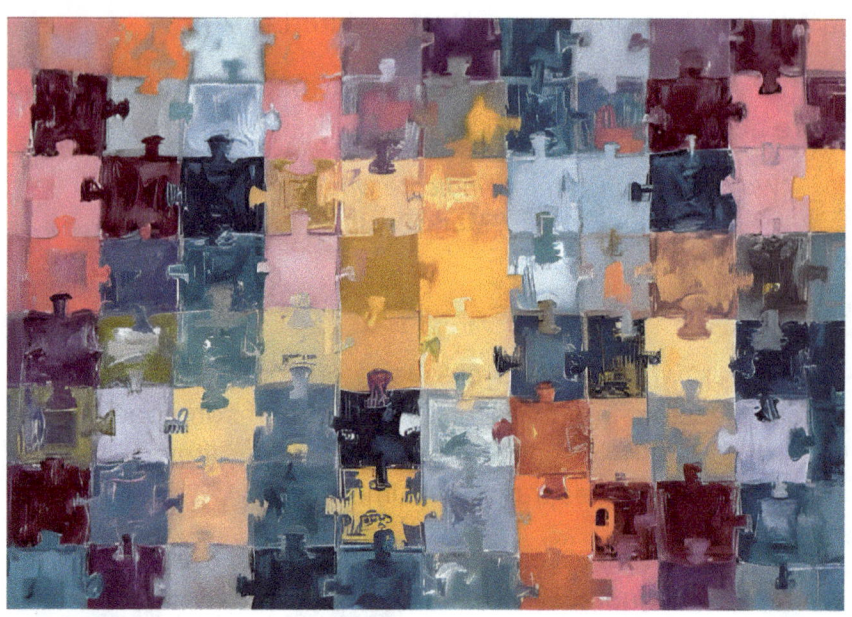

> **Reflection Prompt**

Take a moment to think about your future self, ten or twenty years from now. Imagine looking back at a photo of yourself today. What might you admire about the skin you have right now? What would you wish you had appreciated more in this very moment?

_____
_____
_____
_____
_____
_____
_____

Stories of Kindness

My nana's skin carries the quiet history of a life well-lived. Years in the sun tending her garden left warm freckles and sunspots across her arms. Laughter has carved soft lines around her eyes, the kind that deepen when she smiles. Time has softened her features, her hair now glows silver, but her presence radiates strength, gentleness, and peace.

She is a faithful Christian woman who loves God and her church. Her days have been filled with small joys: sewing quilts with careful hands, piecing together puzzles with patience, and planting flowers that brighten her yard each spring. Her life is stitched together by faith, service, and love, and her skin reflects every moment of it.

When people comment on her beauty, it isn't because her face is free of lines. It's because of the way her eyes light up when she speaks, the kindness in her smile, and the warmth she carries into every room.

Through her, I'm reminded that beauty isn't erased with time. It deepens. True beauty is not the absence of lines, but the presence of a life fully expressed, faithful, and rich with love.

> *"True beauty in a woman is reflected in her soul. It is the caring that she lovingly gives, the beauty of a woman with passing years only grows."* ~**Audrey Hepburn**

The Privilege Mindset

When we view aging as a privilege, every year becomes something to celebrate instead of dread. Instead of asking, *"How do I stop aging?"* we begin to ask, *"How do I live well as I age?"* That change in language transforms anxiety into gratitude.

We begin to see our skin not as betraying us, but as a constant companion through every milestone.

Reflection Prompt

Write down three things you are grateful to have lived long enough to experience. Notice how your skin, in some small way, carries the imprint of those moments. That is beauty worth celebrating.

_____

_____

_____

_____

_____

_____

Life's Roadmap

Aging is inevitable, but fear doesn't have to be. When you recognize that growing older is a gift, you free yourself from the cycle of chasing impossible ideals. You can still protect your skin, nurture your body, and enjoy the journey, but now, you do it with calmness and joy.

The lines on your face are not flaws to erase. They are maps, memories, and proof that you're still here. Aging is not the loss of beauty. It is the deepening of it.

CHAPTER 8

THE GRACE OF GROWING INTO YOURSELF

We've traveled together through the layers of skin, the science of aging, the habits that support resilience, and the myths that cloud our understanding. We've examined how both biology and lifestyle influence the way our skin changes, and we've reframed aging not as something to fear, but as something to be honored.

Now, as we come to the close of this journey, I want to leave you with one final thought: aging is not about losing who you were. It's about becoming more of who you are.

The Balance of Science and Soul

Throughout this book, we've explored the science of skin aging, including collagen, elastin, oxidative stress, hormones, and more. These details matter. They empower us to make informed choices and to protect our skin wisely.

But science alone isn't the whole story. Aging is also an emotional, cultural, and deeply personal experience. It shapes how we perceive ourselves, how others perceive us, and how we interact with the world.

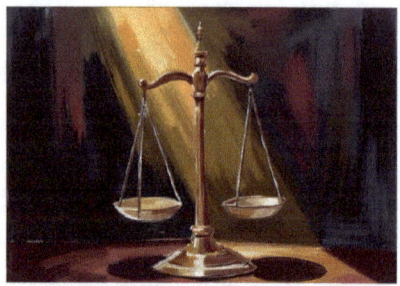

Wrinkles may be rooted in biology, but the meaning we give them comes from our perspective. When we see them as proof of life instead of loss, we restore balance between the outer science and the inner soul.

A Timeless Checklist for Graceful Aging

You don't need complicated routines, endless products, or the latest fads to age with grace. What you need are simple, timeless practices, ones that support both health and happiness.

Protect: Guard your skin with daily sunscreen, gentle care, and barrier support. Protect not just from the sun, but from harsh habits and unnecessary stress.

Nourish: Eat colorful, whole foods. Drink water. Move your body. Choose habits that keep both skin and spirit strong.

Rest: Prioritize sleep, downtime, and emotional balance. Give your body the chance to repair, restore, and renew.

Celebrate: See your skin as a storyteller. Each line, freckle, and mark is a chapter of your life. Celebrate what it reflects.

This checklist is not about perfection. It's about consistency, compassion, and care.

A New Way to See the Mirror

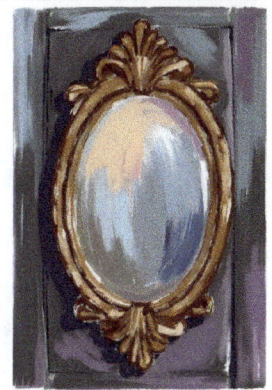

The mirror can be a place of judgment or a place of gratitude. Each time you look at yourself, you have a choice: to see flaws or to see life. To focus on what is "gone," or to honor what remains and what continues to grow.

The next time you catch yourself critiquing a wrinkle or sag, pause and ask, *What does this line represent? What have I lived that gave me this mark?* In that moment, the mirror becomes less of a critic and more of a witness to your journey.

> *"Aging is not about how many years have passed, but how much life you've embraced."*
> ~**Sophia Loren**

Looking Ahead

The beauty of embracing aging is that it opens the door to joy in the present. Instead of anxiously clinging to youth, you can live fully now, nourishing your skin, body, and spirit in ways that make every stage of life meaningful and fulfilling.

Your thirties, forties, fifties, sixties, and beyond are not chapters of decline. They are chapters of becoming. With proper care, your skin can continue to glow, not because it is wrinkle-free, but because it reflects vitality, confidence, and a sense of presence.

Reflection Prompt

Write down three things you want your future self to feel when they look in the mirror. Not how you want to look, but how you want to feel. Maybe it's strong, confident, joyful, or at peace. Let this vision guide the way you care for yourself today.

_____
_____
_____
_____
_____
_____
_____

Closing Words

Aging is universal. It's the most human thing we do. To age is to live, to grow, to deepen. It's a privilege, not a curse.

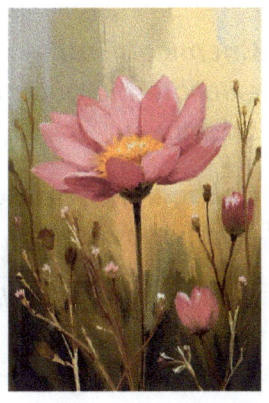

Your skin is not your enemy; it's your companion, carrying you through every season of life. Care for it with knowledge, respect, and compassion. Protect it where you can, accept it where you must, and celebrate it always.

Because the ultimate beauty secret is not eternal youth, it is the grace of growing into yourself.

GLOSSARY OF KEY TERMS

Antioxidants — Compounds (like vitamins C and E) that protect skin cells from damage caused by free radicals, which come from things like UV rays and pollution.

Cell Turnover — The natural process by which old skin cells are shed and replaced with fresh ones. This process slows down as we age, leading to dullness and fine lines.

Ceramides — Fatty molecules naturally found in the skin that strengthen the barrier and help lock in moisture.

Chemical Peel — A professional treatment that uses acids to exfoliate the outer layers of skin, improving texture, tone, and brightness.

Collagen — The main structural protein in the skin that keeps it firm and resilient. Collagen production decreases with age.

Dermis — The middle layer of skin, located beneath the epidermis. It contains collagen, elastin, and blood vessels that provide strength and flexibility.

Epidermis — The skin's outermost layer, acting as a protective shield against the environment.

Exfoliation — The removal of dead skin cells from the skin's surface, either physically (scrubs, brushes) or chemically (AHAs, BHAs).

Extrinsic Aging — Skin changes caused by external factors like sun exposure, pollution, smoking, and lifestyle habits.

Free Radicals — Unstable molecules that damage cells. They are often produced by UV rays, pollution, and stress.

Glycation — A process where excess sugar in the body attaches to proteins like collagen and elastin, weakening them and speeding up skin aging.

Hyaluronic Acid — A molecule naturally found in the skin that holds water, helping keep skin plump, smooth, and hydrated.

Inflammaging — Low-grade, chronic inflammation that develops with age and accelerates skin changes such as wrinkles and loss of firmness.

Intrinsic Aging — The natural aging process determined by genetics and biology, independent of lifestyle factors.

Microneedling — A professional treatment that uses tiny needles to create controlled micro-injuries in the skin, stimulating collagen and elastin production.

Omega-3 Fatty Acids — Healthy fats found in foods like salmon and walnuts that support skin hydration, elasticity, and barrier health.

Oxidative Stress — Cell damage caused by an imbalance between free radicals and antioxidants in the body.

Peptides — Small chains of amino acids that signal the skin to repair itself and produce more collagen and elastin.

Photoaging — Premature aging of the skin caused by repeated sun exposure. It often appears as wrinkles, dark spots, and uneven texture.

Retinoids — Vitamin A derivatives (like retinol) that increase cell turnover, smooth fine lines, and boost collagen.

Skin Barrier — *The outermost part of the epidermis that acts like a wall, keeping moisture in and irritants out.*

Subcutaneous Tissue — *The deepest layer of skin, made of fat and connective tissue that cushions, insulates, and provides structure.*

Sunscreen (Broad-Spectrum) — *A topical product that protects skin from both UVA rays (which cause aging) and UVB rays (which cause burning).*

NOTES:

ALSO BY ASHLYN VAUGHN

If you enjoyed this book, you may also love my other projects designed to bring skincare education, self-care, and creativity into your life:

- **My Skincare Journal: A Cozy Companion for Skincare Tracking, Goal Setting, and Self-Love**
  A guided journal for daily skincare check-ins, progress tracking, and cultivating mindful routines.

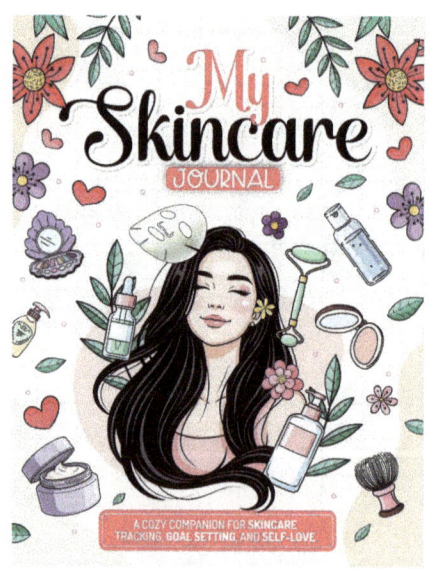

- **The Skincare Word Search Book: Fun & Relaxing Puzzles for Estheticians, Students & Skincare Lovers**
  A playful way to deepen your skincare vocabulary while relaxing.

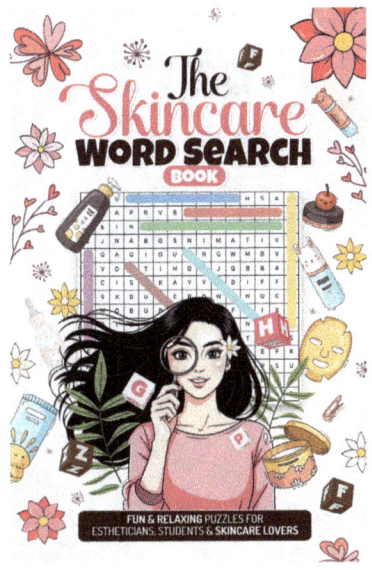

- **The Skincare Crossword Book: Relaxing Crossword Puzzles for Skincare Knowledge & Self-Care Fun**
  Challenge yourself with engaging crossword puzzles centered on skincare science and wellness.

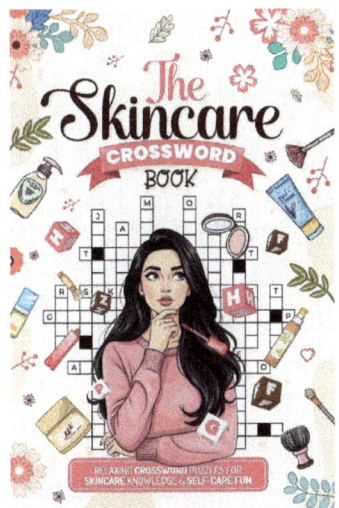

- **Children's Storybook (Theo and Mia's Skin-credible Adventure)** *(Coming Soon)*
  A whimsical journey to teach children about sun safety, hygiene, and the joy of caring for their skin.

  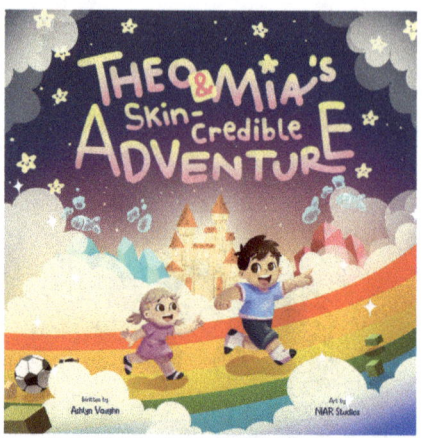

- **Skin Smarts: A Parent's Guide to Children's Skin Health** *(Coming Soon)*
  Practical, science-backed guidance for parents to support their kids' skin with confidence and compassion.

- Explore more of my work and upcoming projects at: https://linktr.ee/skinsmartsofficial

CLOSING NOTE

Thank you for letting this book be part of your journey. If these words inspired you, I would love for you to share your reflections, whether through conversation, journaling, or even an online review. Together, we can shift the way the world views beauty standards and skin aging.

ABOUT THE AUTHOR

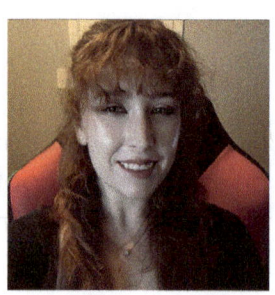

Ashlyn is a native of the Chattanooga, Tennessee area and is a licensed esthetician in the states of Georgia and Tennessee. She graduated from Dalton Institute of Esthetics and Cosmetology in 2021 and has remained committed to continuing her education in skin health.

She has obtained the following service qualifications and certifications:

- Personalized Facials
- Chemical Peels
- Extractions
- LED Therapy
- Microdermabrasion
- Microneedling
- Dermaplaning Certified
- PCA Peel Certified
- Certified Dermalogica Expert
- Certified Hydrafacialist

Having worked at a spa in various capacities—from the front desk to the treatment room—Ashlyn has gained a comprehensive understanding of spa operations. She has also volunteered for a skin & wellness channel, writing online blog posts and contributing to an advice column, *"Ask an Esthetician."* She also participated as a judge in the *2023 SkillsUSA National Esthetics Contest*.

Her work centers on helping others understand the importance of healthy skin habits, whether through practical tools, creative projects, or accessible resources that inspire confidence and consistency. Ashlyn's writing reflects her belief that skincare isn't just a routine, but rather an act of self-love and a lifelong commitment to wellness.

When she's not sharing skincare education, Ashlyn enjoys creating cozy, thoughtful ways for readers to track their progress, reflect on their habits, and find joy in caring for themselves.

content.com/pod-product-compliance
rce LLC
PA
030426
021B/4214